1/2013

With sincere hope of
good journey throug

A Patzer's Journey

Applying the rules from
A Patzer's Story

Timothy A. Sawyer

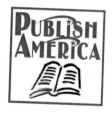

PublishAmerica
Baltimore

First printing

This publication contains the opinions and ideas of its author. Author intends to offer information of a general nature. Any reliance on the information herein is at the reader's own discretion.

The author and publisher specifically disclaim all responsibility for any liability, loss, or right, personal or otherwise, which is incurred as a consequence, directly or indirectly, of the use and application of any contents of this book. They further make no representations or warranties with respect to the accuracy or completeness of the contents of this work and specifically disclaim all warranties including without limitation any implied warranty of fitness for a particular purpose. Any recommendations are made without any guarantee on the part of the author or the publisher.

PublishAmerica has allowed this work to remain exactly as the author intended, verbatim, without editorial input.

Softcover 9781462630271
PUBLISHED BY PUBLISHAMERICA, LLLP
www.publishamerica.com
Baltimore

Printed in the United States of America

This book is dedicated to everyone who has or is currently suffering from depression. It is my sincere hope that all of my books have or will touch you in a positive way.

Preface

The first question to answer is how did I get to this point? Depression is a disease that affects not only myself, but many other people. I can't remember a single event or a single point in life where it started. I can tell you that as the years progressed it was becoming more apparent. Here are my symptoms that led me to believe that I was depressed:

1. Loss of interest in activities
2. Loss of sexual drive
3. Insomnia or inability to stay awake
4. Listlessness
5. Lack of interest in daily work activities
6. Loss of focus
7. Thoughts of suicide

With these symptoms the first step was to see a therapist and get some medication prescribed. This alleviated some of the symptoms but not all of them. For a while I seemed to get better, but over a period of time I was getting steadily worse. The above signs are not all - inclusive.At the beginning of 2010, I was not in a good place because I exhibited all of the above symptoms and more. I had to seek help, and I got the help I needed. **If you suffer from ANY of the above symptoms, PLEASE see your doctor. If you do not have a doctor, talk to someone or go to your nearest hospital emergency room**. Also the website at WebMD.com has numerous resources that you can call on to get the help that you need.

With me being in that condition at the beginning of 2010, I would have laughed if someone had told me that by the end of the year I would be a published author. If you read my first book, <u>A Patzer's Story</u> (ISBN 978-1-4560-3797-0, PublishAmerica, 2010) you would know that 2010 just plain stunk. I was in the midst of a horrible depression where I had to get intensive treatment. Had something inside of me not told me to fight, it is possible that I would not be writing this today. Even though my first book wasn't written until late 2010, it was still written out of frustration. The frustration was brought on by continued losses at the chessboard as well as continued frustration on the bowling lanes, so I felt as though I was stuck. As a form of therapy, I simply started typing… and typing…and typing. Within four days, <u>A Patzer's Story</u> was written. I've taken some heat from reviewers because of that, where the book was lambasted in an early 2011 review because of 'lack of research' and it (my book) being 'only a manifesto'. Call it what you will, but personal reflection requires no research except that of your memories. It was based on my personal experience and contains my opinions. A manifesto? Perhaps. Nevertheless, it was one that helped me. When I wrote the book I had to reflect on my frustrations and why I was feeling frustrated. Once I figured out the "why," then I had to figure out how to overcome them. That is when the rules were developed. The same person who wrote the aforementioned review also said…"what kind of a nut would share his personal journal?" The answer to that is simple. I am the kind of "nut" who wants to share part of his life with others in the hope that if someone reads the book, they would not have to go through what I went through. What's the motivation? Money? No. I said in the book that I had no delusions of <u>A Patzer's Story</u> being on the bestseller list. I had no delusions of a Pulitzer Prize. My motivation was simple; I wanted to give back. Some people these days would find that hard to believe. Believe what you want. I did not go into some details about my personal life. Since I am the author, I get to choose what goes into my books. I also left out personal details to maintain the privacy of people who have been a part of my life. I put in the details that I thought were relevant to the point that I was trying to get across, and even though I know my writing style isn't that of great novelists, I think (with all due modesty) that I did a damn good job.

For reference, here are the rules:

Rule 1: There is no "magic bullet" or "magic pill" that will make you a grandmaster (GM) overnight

Rule 2: You must accept responsibility for your own game and development

Rule 3: What you get out of chess is directly proportional to the effort that you put in

Rule 4: Your opponent is human

Rule 5: Your opponent is out to win and will give you a tough fight

Rule 6: A rating is only a number

Rule 7: Treat your opponent as you want to be treated

Rule 7A: Treat yourself as you want to be treated

Rule 8: Any plan is better than no plan

Rule 9: You may have a plan but your opponent has one too

Rule 10: No plan survives the next move

Rule 11: A chess game is won by the player who makes the NEXT to last mistake[1]

Rule 12: The only game that you should be playing is on the chessboard

Rule 13: Win with grace, lose with dignity

---

1 I am attributing this rule to the two time Polish Chess Champion Savielly Tartakower (1887 – 1956)

Rule 14: Leave your emotions outside the tournament room
Rule 15: Make your opponent EARN the win
Rule 16: Your coach knows more about chess than you do
Rule 17: You learn more when your eyes and ears are open
Rule 18: You learn less when your mouth is open
Rule 19: There is no such thing as a stupid question
Rule 20: Don't let anyone rain on your parade
Rule 21: You must be able to objectively face your current limitations
Rule 22: You must always celebrate and embrace your strengths
Rule 23: There is no such thing as a wrong feeling[2]

I wrote the book from a chess perspective. Hence, a lot of people think it was a book about chess. Yet, if you look at the rules and apply a little imagination, you can surmise that these rules are applicable for almost anything; be it chess, bowling or life itself. While writing and revising the book for publication, the reason for feeling "stuck" became all too clear. The reason I was feeling "stuck" is that I had no "regulation" book to live by. I'm used to regulations. I spent three years in the U.S. Air Force and seven years in the California Army National Guard. If you are currently military or ex-military, you know that the military has a regulation to cover almost everything. I looked at the rules as my little "regulation manual" and vowed to myself that I would strive to follow the rules every day.

This book is about applying the rules in everyday life. There are references to chess and bowling, because these are areas

2 Rule 23 was added with my second book, <u>My Email to God Bounced</u> (ISBN 9781456056278, PublishAmerica, 2011)

that I can relate to as far as the rules are concerned. People have asked me which rule I consider to be the most important, and I find this to be a great question. My answer is that all of the rules are equal in importance, and it also depends on the situation at the moment. Oftentimes I have found that one rule will blend in with another rule. The previous list does not in any way uncover a certain order. Having the rules has at least helped me. I still don't have them memorized, but I can take an experience, look back and say "I applied rule 20" or "that was one for rule 17". For example, take the negative review. At first, yes I was upset. Nonetheless I responded with a rebuttal of sorts, and then in my mind I applied Rule 20 (Don't let anyone rain on your parade). I got published, my books are available world wide and the reviewer didn't present any credentials, so I learned to say "To hell with them", as well as a few other things that are not printable.

Please let me digress with a disclaimer and to clarify something that I mentioned earlier. While this may seem like a personal journal, it is not. I chose to get <u>A Patzer's Story</u> published because I thought it was a valid and pertinient story that needed to be shared, though I only shared those tidbits of my personal life where I felt it was relevant. There are a lot of things in my 48 years that I left out for two reasons; 1) There are some things about myself that I choose to keep private, and I feel that I have the right to do so and 2) There are some things about my life that involved other people and I felt that I had an obligation to protect their privacy. This book will be no different. Where applicable, names of people will be changed and details will be fuzzy. With that, I chose to get this book published for the same reason; I feel that there is value in sharing how these rules have improved my existence and there is a valid and pertnent story to be told. Nonetheless,

I will protect the privacy of those who have been involved with my life and there are simply some things about me that I choose not to disclose to the general public.

I believe in accountability (Rule 2). I also believe in setting the example. It's something like eating your own cooking. When I first wrote the rules, I vowed to make an effort to follow the rules each and every single day. I haven't always done that, but to me that is okay because I'm far from perfect. I know I have limitations (Rule 21), so if something doesn't go as planned I may get a little angry at first, but I know that the anger doesn't really solve the issue. I usually calm down and then look at the issue from a more calmer standpoint. Some of the rules are becoming second-nature. Admittedly, some of the rules are still a challenge. I may not master all of the rules, but I will certainly strive to do so. Even while writing this book which is the "sequel" to my first book, I will be learning things about myself through reflection on my past experiences.

When I started this book, I first started out with the intent of putting the year of 2011 into a "chronicle" of sorts that would give some insight as to how I was applying the rules with different challenges that I have faced. Yet as I was re-writing and revising, I decided to write a chapter on each of the 23 rules with examples of how I applied the rules. To me it is a better form. There are also rules that I will add where appropriate, so chapters will be added for them as well. You will also note throughout the book that I may get "off subject". I may present a rule, explain the context in which I wrote that and then offer a new perspective based on my experiences and reflections over the last several months. While I tend to go on a tangent, I would hope that even the side roads will be fun for you to travel.

I would be remiss if I didn't thank you for reading my book. I don't know why you are reading it, and I don't know where you are at in life. Honestly, I don't need to know. If you have read A Patzer's Story, I want to thank you for reading that too. There is a reason you're reading this book today, but the possible reasons are endless so I won't venture to guess. That is for you to decide. But it is my sincere wish and hope that no matter the reason or your current condition that this book will entertain and possibly enlighten you. More important, it is my hope that I have written something that you can take away with you.

Last but not least, I have added this to each of my other books, and this book will not be an exception. Let me include this quote from My Email to God Bounced:

If you are having thoughts of hurting yourself or others, or if you are thinking about suicide, or if you feel that you are seriously depressed, PLEASE SEEK HELP! Pick up the phone and call 800-273-TALK. This is the number for the National Suicide Prevention Lifeline (www.suicidepreventionlifeline.org*)***. If nothing else, go to your hospital emergency room or call 911.** As I stated in A Patzer's Story your life means something, even if you don't believe it yourself. Let me also state something else; **the help you seek does not come in a bottle, needle or pill.** It comes from people, and it comes from hard work.

By you reading this book, you and I have a connection of sorts. You are learning about me, and what makes me tick. You are also learning what steps I have taken that have been successful with me. Though I don't know anything about you, your struggles or your current condition, let me say this with all sincerity. Your life means something to me. If you read any of my books and can take something away from it that helps you, then my work is done. Helping another person or saving another person's life is worth more than a royalty check.

This is not a 'read this and your life will instantly change' book. I would submit that there is nothing of the sort on this planet. What I will say is that applying the rules will take a lot of hard work and self-reflection on your part. If you strive to apply the rules every day, you will notice a change. The change may be sudden or gradual. Your mileage may vary. It's not going to work all the time. It's not a perfect solution, yet it may give you that extra boost.

As always, I would welcome your feedback. If you have any comments, please contact me via tsawyer@mbdsolus.com or you can vsit my webpage at http://www.authorsden.com/ timothysawyer. Let me leave you with this though through your reading.

It's a good day when you can wake up, accomplish something positive and go to bed knowing that you made your little part of the world a better place. I can't change the world, but if I can make my part better, maybe it will catch on. I do my best to apply the rules on a daily basis

With that, please have a pleasant journey regardless of the road you are on.

Timothy A. Sawyer
March, 2011

Rule 1: There is no "magic bullet" or "magic pill" that will make you a grandmaster (GM) overnight.

To get better at anything takes work and determination. This is true for chess, bowling, your career, or anything. When I first sought therapy for my depression, a therapist gave me a laundry list of books to read. Browsing in my local bookstore, I found books that would claim things like "Depression free in 10 days" or books that would claim to have all the answers to your problems so that your life would be smooth sailing. These books were written by mental health and medical professionals who have more degrees than I have pairs of underwear. I'm not a mental health professional, and have not played one on TV. I don't claim to have the answers, but I am sharing what has worked for me. While I have respect for their education I have a **NEWS FLASH! Live at 11! It's NOT A CURE!** Depression is a life long struggle, at least for me. Therapists that I have seen tend to agree with this. While these books may give you good coping strategies, I need to work to keep my depression in check. When I get up every day, I have to tell myself, at least sub-conciously, that I need to keep my depression in check. That's why I take my medications every day, and I still go to a therapist for on-going maintenance. Don't get me wrong. Books are great, and during my intense therapy we used a lot of excerpts from some great books to drive home points. On the other hand you can do all of the reading that you want to do, but without the application (work) of what you read you will accomplish nothing. I previously stated that the help you seek will take hard work. It's not always easy. In fact, life itself isn't always easy. As you go through whatever process or steps you are taking, there will be bumps in the road. There will be situations that will challenge you. You will have periods of self-doubt and discouragement. Those are the times when you can get strength from other rules in this book. The bottom line is that whatever your pursuits are, whatever your goals are, it takes work and a determination to buckle down and do that work.

How bad do you want it? The answer to this question will gauge your determination. What are you willing to do in order to get what you want? Nobody else can answer that question for you, and sometimes it takes some soul searching. It also sometimes requires some difficult decisions. It sometimes forces you to "step out of the box" or your comfort zone in order to look at things from a different viewpoint. I'll give an example. Last year I was living in New Jersey and bowling regularly. I bowled in a nearby PBA tournament and bowled poorly. After that performance I sought the help of another PBA member who ran the pro shop in one of the houses [3]that I bowled in. He also happens to be a certified coach. So just from these facts alone, we can see that 1) I do not have the natural ability to bowl. This has to be taught and practiced, which takes work. 2) I had (and still have) the determination to put in the effort to improve my game; also note that this ties in with Rule 3, "What you get out of chess is directly proportional to the effort you put in". (By the way, this is an example of a rule blending in with another rule). 3) What I was doing before was not working, as evidenced by my poor performance, so I had to be willing to go outside of my comfort zone to learn new techniques. This also blends in with Rule

3 In bowling parlance, a "house" refers to a bowling center

21, as I was able to face my current limitations. I've always done that but not always with objectivity. My coach showed me some things that I was doing wrong, and pointed out some things that I was doing that I had not even noticed. We had to make some adjustments, and a lot of these adjustments I had never tried before. It took a lot of work and a lot of practice. The results in the beginning were not good, and I was starting to get discouraged. Bear in mind that one of the things that will feed depression is discouragement. If you trust your coach, stick with it. Don't let the discouragement get you down. Gain strength in knowing you had the courage to go into the unknown.

For me, the work that I put into improving my bowling game began to pay off. Although I had to take a break from bowling between September of 2010 and January of this year, I did start to pick up a bowling ball again in January. My results were a little bit slow, but in early April I qualified for the finals in a small tournament. As a result, I finished second in the tournament. There were about 100 entries. I didn't win any money, but it validated a lot of things. For me, it validated that the work and determination will pay off, that you get out what you put in, and there is light at the end of the tunnel.

Rule 2: You must accept responsibility for your own game and development

We hear a lot about 'personal responsibility' and accountability for actions. We have recently seen examples of this where politicians have done really stupid things that have cost them their jobs. I myself have done many stupid things, and I have owned up to them. In some cases I am still paying the price. The stupid things that I have done would be the subject of another book, in several volumes that would take me a long time to write and would fill at least one entire bookshelf, if not the Library of Congress. Yes, we must accept responsibility for our actions, and sometimes it isn't easy to do. Nevertheless there is a fine line between accepting responsibility and dwelling on them to the point where it becomes detrimental. This has been my problem in that I focused too much on the mistakes that I made in my past. This was a contributor to the "downward spiral" that caused my depression. In chess, once you make a move you can't take it back. If it is a bad move, you learn from it. If it is a good move, that's okay. In both cases though, it happened and you can't change it. We all sometimes wonder what it would be like to go back in time and undo the mistakes that we made, and while it is a good thought, it is impossible in today's world. So while we must accept responsibility and be held accountable, we must also be able to accept the fact that it can't be undone. While we must face our mistakes, we must also be able to learn from them and keep moving forward. Don't dwell on the past, especially when the past brings back bad memories. This type of dwelling has thrown me into downward spirals. Please don't let that happen to you.

Rule 2 also goes beyond accountability. The real intent behind this rule was to emphasize the importance of taking a leadership role in your development for whatever improvement that you would seek. There is a saying out there somewhere that says, "If you want to do something right, do it yourself". If you're sitting on a couch, in a funk and taking no action to get yourself out of the funk, you're not taking a leadership role, and from outward appearances you're not determined to put in the work to help yourself. If the determination isn't there, that is certainly your choice but you also have to be aware that there are consequences to action or even inaction. I myself have been guilty of inaction, and in some cases it has cost me dearly. To this day and for a time to come, the inaction that I chose to exercise recently will cost me in the future. I've accepted that, I've accepted the consequences so now I move on as best as I can.

Early in 2010, I was in such a depressed state that I couldn't work. I couldn't concentrate and I couldn't focus. It was difficult just to get out of bed sometimes. I had no choice but to take a leave of absence from my job so that I could seek treatment. My doctor put me on antidepressants, and it was up to me to find a therapist as well as a psychiatrist. The first therapist that I had didn't really impress me. We didn't seem to hit it off, so after two visits I sought out another therapist as well as a psychiatrist. While I clicked more with these providers, I could only see them weekly, if I was lucky. Since I wasn't working, this left me alone and with much time on my hands to do nothing. The only thing that I did on a regular basis was bowl, and that probably was the only thing that held me together - as I didn't have Wendy, who is my nine-year old Shih-Tzu that I adopted in early May. Having much time to do nothing was dangerous. I wasn't making any progress and I was slipping. I had to take charge, and insist on an emergency appointment with my psychiatrist to explain to her what was going on. Only then did she finally get me into intensive outpatient treatment. This turned out to be the catalyst that helped me turn the corner.

A leadership role means that you are involved in your process of getting better. I took a leadership role in seeking out a different approach in handling my depression. To me, though, this did not mean that I walked into therapy on day one and started to tell my therapists and staff that I knew more than they did. My therapist and all the staff people involved with my treatment had degrees and training in mental health treatment. I do not. My therapist and all the staff people involved with my treatment had experience in dealing with depression. I did not. This is rule 16, "Your coach knows more about chess than you do". In my opinion, a good leader forms a team of people who have skill sets in different areas, and figures out a way to make all the skill sets complementary to accomplish the mission. While I didn't get to choose my therapist, I was blessed to have this sort of team of people to work with. This doesn't mean that you get to kick back while they do the work. This was especially true in therapy. I had to work for it. I had to share things about my life that I never shared with anyone. There were many tears, many fears and much anxiety. I listened, I participated and I tried to see things in a different light. Sometimes it didn't always work but for the most part, my therapy turned on the light. This is because I was willing to put in the work, and I was willing to take a leadership role, but at the same time willing to let my therapist and staff do their jobs.

One of the character flaws that I still have is stubbornness. This doesn't work well in therapy. My mother, and my grandmother before her are very set in their ways. I remember my grandmother having the same breakfast every morning. I remember her having almost the same dinner every night. My mother, to a point was very set in her ways. When I was growing up, every Saturday was house cleaning day, with few exceptions. So while I get my stubbornness honestly, it doesn't work well when you're trying to get better in any endeavor. When I was getting my coaching last year, I had to really work to put my stubbornness away and try something new. The old way wasn't working, but it's what I knew. In therapy, I really had to step out of the box and try new things. It's scary but I tried. Yes, I can still be stubborn and it shows today. Then again, remember with any endeavor, you have to be flexible to change.

The other point behind Rule 2 is the keyword "You". You have to take a leadership role. Now I mentioned earlier that the people involved in your development have the training and skill sets to help you, yet you must be wary of 'unsolicited' advice that can come from family, friends or acquaintances. Remember this - nobody knows your situation better than you. People generally mean well, but this can derail your own progress so take this advice sparingly. Don't give in to negative influences about your progress. This applies if your own conscious is the influence or if there are other outside influences. These influences WILL derail your progress.

Rule 2 has many different connotations, yes. The key words to remember are responsibility, leadership and most importantly, YOU!

Rule 3: What you get out of chess is directly proportional to the effort you put in

This is a culmination of the first two rules, so I won't belabor this. If you're willing to work, and you accept responsibility for what you have to do, you are going to put in a good amount of effort to get where you want to be. The more effort you put in, the more potential return you will get out of it. With my therapy, this was so true. I'll tell you what didn't happen. I didn't sit around and let someone prescribe antidepressants, hoping I would get better. Nobody was handing me a magic cure. While it is an effort to take the medication, it is not the 'end all, be all'. Trust me on that one. Nobody is going to hand you anything. Nobody is going to hand you a book, and tell you that if you put it under your pillow, all of your wishes will come true. This isn't the tooth fairy we are discussing. This is life. Nobody handed me anything. I was expected to show up for my therapy sessions and participate. This means that I had to put in effort. The effort I put in helped me turn the corner. After therapy, and after I started to feel better, I couldn't say enough good things about the help that I got. In spite of this I had one friend tell me, "You did it". At first I shrugged it off, but it's true. I did do it. I had help, but I did it. There are a few examples where I have already illustrated where this rule applies, but I will share a couple more.

At the beginning of the year, I entered a chess tournament to be played by email. The format was a seven player section, which turned out to be one game against each of the other six players. In my previous correspondence tournament, I withdrew from it since it was at the height of my depression, but I wanted to get back into it. It turns out that two of the players were people that I faced in my last tournament so I knew I was in for at least a couple of tough games. Now with correspondence chess, you are allowed to consult printed matter (books, magazines, etc.) but not other players or use computer engines (though you can use computers for record keeping). The chess lessons that I got helped. I'll share one of the games (the name of my opponent was changed for the sake of privacy). If you are unfamiliar with chess notation, I included a short tutorial at the end of the book. You can also drop me an email for more information.

[Event "USCF 11ET02 Express Tournament"]
[Site "Correspondence"]
[Date "2011.01.16"]
[Round ""]
[White "Sawyer, T"]
[Black "Mark"] (Name changed for privacy)
[ECO "E00"]
[Result "1-0"]
1.d4 Nf6 2.c4 e6 3.g3 Bb4+ 4.Nd2
c5 5.a3 Bxd2+ 6.Qxd2 cxd4 7.Bg2 Nc6
{And not 7. Qxd4? which loses a tempo to 7....Nc6. The doubled pawns on Black's d-file is good compensation for the loss of a pawn}
8.Nf3 b6 9.Nxd4 Bb7
{So here I have taken back the pawn and gained a definite space advantage at the center. I would love to exploit Black's weakness at c7 by getting my Knight on there with a fork but I would expect Black to castle short. I also need to make my King safe and get my dark B into play so that should be a priority.}

10.e4 Nxd4 {e4 is better than 0-0 because this is a direct challenge to the center}

11.Qxd4 h6 12.Bf4 O-O 13.Bd6 Re8

{As it turned out, 13. Bd6 becames Black's downfall because it took control of two major diagonals and really cramped Black}

14.O-O {Black resigns} 1-0

Trust me, this was a tough game. It looked easier than it really was. I had to check and double check each move to make sure that it was the best move I can find. The key was that I didn't rush my moves.

The rest of the tournament was the best result I had in a while, four wins and two draws. One win was by forfeit (my opponent never sent a move) while another was my opponent resigning after one move because he realized that he didn't have the time for the game. In spite of this, two wins (this and another game) were good games with tough fights.

Another example of effort happened recently. In the midst of writing this book, I entered an Over The Board (OTB) tournament. It spanned a weekend, and even though the drive was sometimes long I thought it was worth it. So beforehand, I did as much preparation as I could with notes, online resources, computer, and whatever I had at my disposal. Admittedly, I didn't have much time to prepare but I did what I could. I will talk some more about this in the next chapter, but the tournament result was not bad at all with two wins, two losses and one draw. All the players except one (and he put up a good fight) were rated higher than me. The truth is that the effort that I put into preparing, as well as the effort that I put into my tournament games paid dividends. The effort that I put into my therapy paid dividends. Effort begets dividends.

There is something else that I learned over the months that is not yet a rule - but will be. I was diagnosed with a herniated disc in my neck that was the culprit of my shoulder problems. I was referred to a pain management doctor who recommended a cortisone shot in my neck. I have had them in my shoulders, and they can be somewhat uncomfortable, but getting one in my neck - close to my spinal cord - made me a little nervous. Despite that, I went ahead and scheduled the procedure. On the day of the procedure, I was placed on an examination table with a huge X-ray machine, used so that the doctor could pinpoint where the needle needed to go. It was uncomfortable, but I thought that a little discomfort now was worth the result. So on an examination table, having a needle placed in my neck gave me the inspiration for Rule 24 - "A little discomfort is sometimes necessary to achieve the desired result". As I thought about this and looked back, this was also true of my therapy as well as the "funk" that inspired me to write my first book. Going through therapy was uncomfortable and sometimes downright emotionally draining. Yet when I look back at where I was then compared to where I am today, it was worth the pain and discomfort. The key to Rule 24 is that when you feel the discomfort or pain, you have to keep your eye focused on the goal. If the pain becomes unbearable, then it is time to reevaluate, because constant pain is not a good thing.

You get out what you put in. That's the gist of this rule. It ties back to the willingness to work, or the determination to put in the effort. The determination also includes the ability to withstand the discomfort that may accompany the effort. Don't lose sight of where you want to end up.

Rule 4: Your opponent is human,
Rule 5: Your opponent is out to win and will give you a good fight,
Rule 6: A rating is only a number

I decided to put rules 4, 5 and 6 in the same chapter because they are very much related as they deal with opponents. Also, rule 6 has some different connotations that I will share. When I wrote these rules, I was reflecting on my (then) recent chess games. I wasn't really considering the overall connotations of the rules themselves. Now, as I read and reflect on the rules, I am going to make some corrections.

Rule 4 says, "Your opponent is human". On reflection, this is not always true. As well as human opponents, there are also opponents that are inanimate. The true definition of an inanimate opponent is very subjective and depends on the situation. For example, a golfer would view the course or the different holes on the course as being opponents, with the unpredictability of the slope of the grass, the placement of the sand traps and even the placement of the hole. For bowlers, it could be the lanes, with the unpredictability of the oil patterns and how each lane reacts differently. The inanimate opponent has characteristics that you can't see and it can't see you.

I've said throughout my books, and talking to people that depression is the toughest opponent I have ever faced, tougher than any person I have met across a chessboard. Depression is not a human opponent, though it does affect humans. Nonetheless, it is a tough opponent that I face every day. I accept the fact that I will not win every chess game I play, or will I bowl consecutive 300 games. I accept the fact that I will lose arguments and that I will not always get my way, but what I will never do is resign to depression. I do not ever again want to be in a state that I was last year. For me to know depression, I had to face it. I couldn't see it but it was attacking me internally. Once I faced it I could see the characteristics and combat them. To do that, I had to face it. I couldn't turn a blind eye to it any longer. Once I knew what it was, I could do something about it. To overcome an opponent, you must face the opponent. Whether the opponent is human or inanimate, you must face it, which is the first step in winning.

Also on reflection, Rule 5 and Rule 6 tie together nicely but let me make a further observation on Rule 5. On the chessboard, all of my opponents, win or lose have given me good games and put up tough fights. Rule 5 will always holds true for a human opponent. What about the inanimate opponents? A bowling lane has no ego, nor does a golf course have drive or a will to win. Hence, they are not out to beat you. The only way that you can lose to an inanimate opponent is to beat yourself. In the 32 years that I have been bowling, I have been guilty of blaming the lanes for poor performance. I can't tell you how many times I have heard the same from other bowlers. My exposure to the level of competition in the PBA has taught me one thing, which is that the lane didn't beat me. Granted, there are some pairs[4] of lanes that are tougher than others, and lanes may not be consistent from house to house. Notwithstanding, I beat myself. I beat myself by not paying attention and adjusting to the lane condition. I failed to take responsibility (Rule 2) and a leadership role. It's that simple. This realization is not meant to be self-deprecating, and it is

---

4 Sanctioned bowling competition takes place on a pair of lanes where each frame is bowled on an alternate lane

void of emotion, which is Rule 21 - Being able to objectively face your current limitations. It is still a simple reality. I've had to adopt the same attitude with my depression. If I let it consume me, I'm done. Beating me when it comes to my depression is a far worse loss than any loss that I may suffer at the chessboard.

I understand that this all seems extremely simplistic. Trust me when I say that it is not as simple as it looks on paper - far from it. The path to get from where I was at the beginning of 2010 to where I am at today has been a tough, emotional road filled with pot holes and speed bumps. Moving forward, I am equally certain that there are more speed bumps ahead. Half of the battle is being able to navigate the pot holes, speed bumps and sharp corners but it can be done. Yes, reading it here makes it seem all too easy. A couple of weeks ago I was bowling in one of my regular leagues and had a particularly good game. One of the bowlers on the opposing team said to me, "You make it look so easy". I have heard that before, and writing this reminded me of it. When everything flows well, yes it looks so easy. It flows well when I have my mind focused on the task at hand, but even then it is not as easy as it looks. Once I lose focus, I become frustrated and intimidated, thinking that I can never do this. The same thing happens at a chessboard when I sit across from someone who has a much higher rating than I do, which happened at the recent tournament I referenced earlier. In the first game, I thought that I was going to have my face used to clean the chessboard and have pawns stuck up my nose but that wasn't the case. What I did was to focus on playing the best game possible and I ended up winning that game. On the opposite end of the spectrum are being too complacent, taking things for granted. At the same tournament, I was paired up against a player who had a lower rating than I did. Did I take that for granted? Certainly not, as he played a good game, and though I won it was a tough game. While "A rating is only a number" was really written with an emphasis on chess, the bigger picture behind this rule is that with enough focus and determination, any opponent can be overcome no matter how daunting the odds are.

A chess rating is a measure of a person's relative playing strength. In other words, a player with a 2000 rating should usually beat a player with a 900 rating. Conversely, I have beaten players with a higher rating, and I have also lost games to those with a lower rating. When I started writing <u>A Patzer's Story</u>, I was getting beaten. As I wrote more, I realized that it wasn't just at the chessboard. I looked at my obstacles as huge barriers that I couldn't overcome. Physically, I was having shoulder issues. Mentally, I was worried about business. I was stuck. I felt like I was sinking back into a depression, which prompted me to write the book. After writing it, I took a step back. I started to break down my obstacles into smaller, more manageable challenges. The point here is that an obstacle or opponent can be overcome, regardless of its strength.

Taking Stock: Rules 1 - 6

I thought this would be a good place to take a deep breath and take stock. Focus, determination, work, responsibility and leadership were all key words in the first few sections. You may be starting to think that it is sounding like one of those self-help seminars where the speaker was down to his last two quarters and turned it into a million dollars within the year. "Just do this, and this, and this. Oh by the way buy this and this for more insight..." and your problems will be solved. I can tell you that this book is not like that. As I stated before, there is no cure for depression; at least from what I can tell; and reading this book does not guarantee you smooth sailing. No book in the world is a substitute for the determination and work that it took me to get to the point where I am today. It simply does not work that way.

I'm not going to say that my life has been hard or cruel. To look back and blame my upbringing or my childhood or my marriages for what has taken place is just an excuse. Make no mistake that my life has gone over tough roads. I've been married and divorced three times. It takes two to make a marriage work, and I didn't do my part. Many of the things that I have been through were quite frankly, self-inflicted by my own irresponsibility and ignorance. Some of the things that I have been through were due to circumstances beyond my control. All of that adds up to what my life has been, and what leads me here today. I didn't write A Patzer's Story or this book to seek pity. I don't want pity, I don't deserve pity and quite frankly I don't need it. Unfortunately though, there are some people who thrive on it. Pity, in my opinion, breeds an illusion that all you have to do is sit back, let other people do the work for you and either it will get better, or if it doesn't, you can blame those who did the work. If people want to live like that it is their choice but it is not the choice that I made. I have made choices in my life, some good, some worse and some just downright horrible. On the other hand a good choice that I made is not accepting pity from those that offered it. While they have good intentions, pity is not what I need.

What I do need, and what I strive for, is the determination to make the effort everyday to keep my depression in check. It is an opponent that will never be beaten, but it is one that can be held back. It's almost like the Demilitarized Zone at the 38th Parallel that separates North Korea from South Korea. Technically, these two nations are still at war but a truce keeps the two countries from a shooting war. Yes, there are skirmishes along the border, and much saber rattling, but there is still a sense of peace, albeit tense. My depression is a good parallel to this. Though there is no truce, my determination and my effort will keep my depression at its borders. That is what I strive for every day.

Rule 7: Treat your opponent, as you want to be treated,
Rule 7A: Treat yourself as you would want to be treated

Sound familiar? Respect by others is a basic human need, according to Abraham Maslow (A Theory of Human Motivation, A.H. Maslow, 1943). Hence, we all want to be treated with courtesy and kindness. I will go even farther and say that everyone deserves to be treated with courtesy and kindness. Sometimes it isn't returned and that can be a little disturbing but that shouldn't keep us from practicing it. Rule 7 is probably the rule that I am most conscious of. I don't always follow it, but I try. I sometimes don't follow it when someone cuts me off on the road. Even though I live in Kentucky now, I still use the New Jersey turn signal (honk on the horn followed by extended middle finger), and that isn't exactly kind or courteous. Again, I'm not perfect. Not everyone treats me with kindness or courtesy, either. While it bothers me, it didn't bother me as much as it did before. I used to take many things personally. I had very low self-esteem and I really wanted people to like me, because I wasn't well liked; or I perceived that I wasn't well liked. I didn't have many friends when I was growing up, and this was probably by choice. I was used to doing things alone and finding ways to entertain myself, but back then it was really tough for me to take rejection and it was even tougher for me to treat myself with kindness.

Before I got my PBA card, I think that bowling was a chore because I was really hard on myself and I didn't cut myself much slack. I wasn't very personable, I didn't talk with many people and I think that my reputation was somewhat of a real jerk. Many people were afraid to approach me because they didn't know how I would react. Looking back, I don't blame them. I wasn't treating myself very well, so how should I be expected to treat others with kindness? It wasn't just bowling and chess where I would habitually beat myself up. I didn't have much confidence in myself, so I expected perfection every time, and on reflection this was an attempt to bolster my own self-esteem. I threw myself in any endeavor I took seriously, whether it was work, bowling or chess. I didn't want to do anything halfway and I still don't. I still beat myself up, sometimes. Lately though, I have been trying to give myself a break and look at things with a "glass half full" attitude. This attitude has helped me to look at people in a different, more positive light.

My attitude has also helped me see just how hurtful, negative and downright mean some people are. In life, there are positive and negative forces. No matter where you go or what you do, there is always some sort of negative force nearby whether it is a person or a situation. You just have to decide what is positive for you, what is negative for you and figure out how you're going to deal with it. In theory, this is simple but in practice it is difficult. In life, positive and negative forces are subjective. What one sees as positive, another may see as negative. The decision of what is positive and negative in your life and surroundings is yours and yours alone. Once you make that decision, the manner in which you confront or ignore it is also up to you. Without revealing content, I got a nasty email from someone earlier this year. It was one of the first emails I saw that morning, and I was taken aback by it. When I read it, I was kind of in shock. My first impulse was to immediately reply with a scathing email of my own, but then I had to stop and consider that. A "knee jerk" reaction would usually get me into trouble, and I didn't want to say anything I would regret. I decided to leave the email alone for a while until I felt that I could formulate a reply. A week later, I did reply to the email. I stated the facts as I saw them, and outlined my proposed resolution. I thought it was a well written email, void of any name calling or accusations (except where I referred to the original email as unprofessional). The email I received in return was professional, and although differences still remain, I said nothing that I would regret and I think that with some negotiation the differences can be worked out. Despite the negative tone of the original email, I managed to apply Rule 7 and things seemed to work out. What I learned from this experience is that applying negative to negative only yields negative. Remember basic math:$-2 + (-2) = -4$ and $-2 - (-2) = 0$. When I am negative, I go into my downward spiral. If I apply a positive to a negative, I turn toward or stay positive which helps my psyche. It may not change the situation or the person. In A Patzer's Story I cautioned about those things that you have no control over. What you do have control over is your reaction.

Despite all my efforts to maintain a positive spin and to be positive with other people, it still pains me to see how brutally negative people can be, and the effect it has on other people. It pains me even more to see these negative people have the attitude that nothing is wrong with them. This is why no matter what, I always try to be positive, courteous and friendly to all those I come in contact with. Do I sometimes fail? Yes, but there are some occasions when a lack of courtesy is warranted but these are few and far in between. I have found that being positive, courteous and friendly helps my overall outlook because no matter how someone acts toward me, I know that I have taken the high ground and I feel better about myself. I actually, in a way, feel sorry for those people who choose to be negative. Their positive seems to be our negative. Unfortunately, the negativity isn't contained and spills over, which affects innocent people. Like the weather, we have no control over it but the effect is far-reaching. I know it is wishful thinking for these people to drop the negativity. It pains me to see it, and I'm sure it pains other people. For me, the best way to not let it affect me is to stay clear away from it, surround myself with positive people and positive influence as much as possible and to try to live my life in a positive manner each day.

Rule #7 not only applies to 'opponents' but to people who are not your opponents. I'll be the first to admit that I don't always follow this rule. If someone cuts me off on the road, doesn't use their turn signal or does other stupid things, I may shake my head in disgust, question their parentage or call them names under my breath. Again, I'm not perfect. It pains me though to see people in their own little world with little or no regard for others. One night, I was driving to the bowling alley. I was on a city street, and an older man was trying to negotiate the sidewalk in his electric wheelchair. As I was passing him, he literally fell over as he hit a rut in the sidewalk. I couldn't stop there, but after a quick thought I turned around and went back. There he was, standing, (fortunately unhurt) with his wheelchair on the side. He couldn't pick it up. I picked it up, set it upright, helped him get in it and he was on his way. Nobody else stopped to even see if he was okay. I would hate to think how long he would be there until someone gave him some assistance. I open the door for people, or hold it open if someone is behind me. If I have a lot of stuff at the grocery store and the person behind me has only a few things, I let them ahead of me in line. It's the little things like that which can not only make your day better, but help you to feel better. These little things truly make a difference in other people's lives. Very recently, my neighbor was having a problem getting his truck started. He and a friend of his were trying to clean up the battery terminals. I suggested baking soda, which he didn't have. So I went into my house, mixed a solution of baking soda and water, then grabbed a wire brush from my gun cleaning kit. I helped him clean the terminals, and a few minutes later he was able to get his truck started. He asked, "How much do I owe you?" I replied, "Nothing." He looked at me quizzically and asked, "You sure?" I said, "Just a neighbor helping a neighbor"

Something as simple as 1/4 cup of baking soda with tap water in a jar and a $.59 wire brush can make a difference in someone's day.

I'm sure that the gentleman in the wheelchair has forgotten about me, but I was able to make his day a little more positive. My neighbor will go on about his business, and not give it a second thought. I'm okay with that, because the objective of rule #7 is not only to treat your opponent with dignity and courtesy, but also to try in some way to make a small difference in the lives of people around us. If my writings can accomplish this, then that is the epitomy of rule #7.

Deep Breath

All of these rules came to me as a result of self-analysis and reflection. I can't explain how they came to me, except that they just popped into my head as I was thinking about different things or in some cases, stewing about different things. Some of these even hit me before I started writing A Patzer's Story. So I can't explain the how. There were, and still are, many "AHA!" moments; one of those moments where the light bulb finally comes on. I'm a work in progress. I'm not perfect, nor will I ever be. All I can do, and all I can ever be asked to do is try my best. Whatever I do, whatever I undertake, I give it all my energy. This is true for chess, bowling, my therapy, my job, and anything that I am involved with and that I feel a passion for. Until I published A Patzer's Story, I never thought that I would have a passion for writing. I've been told that I have a gift for it, but I never believed it. Then again, as people started to see my books and comment on them, I was surprised to see how many people told me that they could relate to me. I've said this before, but I will say it again. If one life is touched, changed for the better or if because of my writings I can help pull someone from the brink of despair, that is worth more than a royalty check. I may never know how many lives have changed because of my writing. Maybe it is a leap of faith that people have read my book and had an "AHA!" moment of their own. Maybe it is this leap of faith, and a true passion to help others that has kept me writing and not giving up when it seemed hopeless.

Rule 8: Any plan is better than no plan, Rule 9: You may have a plan but your opponent has one too, Rule 10: No plan survives the next move

Like Rule 7 and 7A, these rules are interrelated. If you have no plan when playing a chess game, your chances of winning the game are extremely slim. If you have no plan in your life, your chances of winning are extremely slim. Now I am going to contradict myself and say that nobody has "no plan" or the corollary that is "Everyone has a plan". We all have a plan. The difference, besides the goal, is the extent of the plan. The goal in mind may be to eat some food. We all have to eat, so we all would plan how we would reach that goal. The differences in the plan are countless, but there is still a plan. While most people will have a plan for basic survival (food, clothing and shelter), there are some people that don't have a plan for higher ambitions, such as relationships, career or anything else. This is because they are struggling with basic survival. If someone is at that point in their life, it is almost impossible to strive for higher goals. At one time or another, many of us have been there. When I was going through therapy, and for a while after, I was just trying to make it day by day with no eye toward the future. My mantra was "Just get me through another day of getting better". I wasn't thinking about the next year, month or in some cases even the next day. I was thinking about basic survival. I had food, I had clothing and I had shelter, but I just wanted to get through the day without breaking down. There were days when getting out of bed was a major milestone. We all have a plan in some form. How extended that plan is, or what the goals are varies from person to person. There were some days when I didn't feel as though I had a plan, but subconsciously I really did.

I know quite a few people who have panic attacks about plans. I used to be one of them. If everything was planned to the most minor detail, even one detail changed in the slightest, I felt out of sorts. On the other extreme, I know people who just fret about having a plan. What's the right thing to do? What if this goes wrong? What if that goes wrong? They work themselves to a point where they are panicking about having a plan, and don't get anything accomplished. Just do it. Any plan is better than no plan. We are never 100% certain if a plan will work. I've been stuck in that situation too. Just execute.

Having a plan has risks. There have been many times when I have had a plan to do something, and it gets derailed, or I have a plan to do something and something changes where I would have to change plans on the fly. Rules 9 & 10 are very interrelated, and that is where this comes into play. I can't count how many chess games I have played where I would make a move with a specific plan in mind, and all of a sudden my opponent would either thwart me with a plan I did not see, or my opponent does something totally unexpected where a new plan is possibly uncovered. It works both ways, positive and not so positive. When I started to feel better, I found that my plans went beyond the daily survival. I started planning for my business. I started thinking about a more permanent home. I started thinking about some higher ambition plans. Accomplishing a goal based on a plan helped boost my self confidence. Getting my first and second books published were part of a plan, and now I'm bouncing ideas around for my fourth book.

Also tightly intertwined with Rules 8, 9 and 10 are goals and goal setting. A goal is the desired result of a plan. I did talk about goals in A Patzer's Story but a recent experience that I had will really drive this whole point home. So I'm going to exercise some literary license and go off on a tangent. In my first book, I talked a lot about chess but not a lot about my second passion, bowling. At the time I wrote A Patzer's Story, I wasn't bowling because of a shoulder problem. In spite of this, I have since started bowling again so I thought that in a discussion about goals and plans I would share this.

I was not athletically inclined when I was growing up. I didn't play Little League, Pop Warner or any other sports. Some would have called me a klutz back then, and after review I would agree with them. When I was a sophomore in high school, someone suggested that I join the bowling club. I did, and became hooked on the sport. Now remember that starting out, I wasn't very good. I even continued to bowl when I was in the Air Force but stopped before I got out. I never lost the love for bowling though. When a friend invited me to join his bowling league some years later, I did. I guess you could say that I got "re-hooked". It was a slow process. I bowled whenever I got the chance. My dream in high school was to get on a TV show like the PBA pros. That dream never went away. I practiced, practiced and practiced, took lessons, new bowling balls - the works. Finally in the mid 1990s I felt like it was coming together. In 1997 I did qualify to join the Professional Bowler's Association (PBA) but since I was moving from CA to the East Coast I didn't put in my application. When I got to the East Coast, I bowled again, but it was not the same as when I was in CA. I struggled for a few years, but finally in 2005 it all came together. In late 2005, I got a postcard from the PBA promoting a membership special. Let me digress here for a moment; in 1997, one of the membership requirements for the PBA was a 200+ average over the two previous seasons, which I qualified for in 1997. Yet, in 2005 I was well short of that. Unknown to me, until I looked on their website in 2005, they had changed that requirement to a 200 average in 36 games. I certainly did that in 2005. Figuring a 50 / 50 chance of being accepted, I sent my application to the PBA. It was accepted, and now the dream is almost reality. Instead of the dream though, I got an education in reality. Bowling in league is nothing close to bowling in a PBA tournament. Since my first tournament in 2006, I generally have not fared well, which has contributed to my frustration and discouragement.

After a tournament in July 2010, the arthritis and tendonitis in my shoulder had me to the point where I couldn't bowl. Hence, I didn't pick up a bowling ball until January of this year. When I did finally start bowling on a regular basis again I had to reeducate myself. Not so much in the physical aspect, but the mental aspect. I had to cut myself some slack because it had been a while since I bowled. Overall, I was doing okay. The pain in the shoulder was minimal, and my bowling was okay. In mid-March, the center where I bowled sponsored a charity tournament in April. Free entries to the finals were being given to those who scored well enough in the "house qualifier", where you would use your scores from a regular league night. One league night I entered and bowled well enough to qualify for the finals in early April. I bowled two squads in the finals, and in my second squad shot a three-game 670 series. This was good enough for second place. I didn't win any money (which wasn't my aim) but what a confidence builder. The difference, I think, between this recent tournament and other past tournaments is that I didn't over plan and I didn't set huge expectations. I'm very, very guilty of over planning. To me, over planning is making a plan to such a degree that when the circumstances or conditions change, I'm lost. Being lost contributes to a downward spiral.

Before this last tournament in March, I would take any chess tournament or bowling tournament very seriously. If it were a bowling tournament I would practice, practice and practice some more. I would work myself into such a mental frenzy that when the tournament grew closer, nothing else really mattered. Mental game experts would tell you to "visualize". I did that a lot. I felt that if I visualized myself getting that trophy, nothing would stop me. What I didn't realize before recently was that I was mentally setting myself up for failure. Winning became the goal and not the dream. I was clouding what was realistic with what was out of my control. If I didn't attain the goal of winning the tournament, I went into a downward spiral. Winning was not a realistic goal, because I had no control over what the other players bowled. In March, I had the goal of just bowling the best that I could. The same could be said for my recent chess tournament. I just went there and played the best I could play.

Any plan is better than no plan. The more realistic the goal, the easier it is to achieve. The more goals you are successful at, the better you feel about yourself. The more flexible you are with changing circumstances, the easier it is to adapt your plans to meet the change. This has been a tough set of lessons for me to learn.

Whatever your plan is, whether it is to get better at some endeavor, or just a plan to make it through the day, I wish you success. A plan achieved is a step toward victory.

Rule 11: A chess game is won by the person who makes the NEXT to last mistake

"How could they do that?"

"How did they let that happen?"

"Why did I do that? I didn't see that!"

How many times have we seen a mistake by a sporting team only to get the win because their opponent made a mistake at the end? All the previous mistakes are nullified because of that final mistake. The end result is a win, so all of the previous errors are history. But make that last mistake, and everything else that was done right is lost in the clutter. In chess games, it doesn't matter if you drop a Bishop and win the game. Conversely if you're up a Bishop and make a glaring blunder which loses the game, that becomes the perennial focus. I've been on both sides of the table. I've made the last mistake, and I've made the next to the last mistake. I've made more of the "last mistakes" then the "next to last mistakes". To be honest, I don't remember what brought on this rule, except that I was thinking about all of the games that I lost and dwelling on the "mistakes" that my opponent made that I didn't see. As I was preparing to write this book I took out the rules and reflected on each one of them to be able to relate personal experiences. I reflected on this one for quite a while, and I'll admit a bit of "writers block" because I really didn't know how to proceed. On reflection, this is a very important rule to dwell on.

Humans make mistakes. I make them, you make them. Some are big, some are small. Some only cause a little discomfort and some cause a lifetime of change. They are made because of knowledge or lack of knowledge, and choices. I've made mistakes because of bad choices. I've made mistakes because I "didn't know any better". That's where I would get stuck and get caught in the downward spiral. I would try to examine the "Why". My favorite questions to myself are "How could I have been so stupid?", "How could I do such a thing?" and others that are not printable. The "why" was followed with a pretty good character assasination of myself by me. Nobody does a better job of beating me down than me, but that still didn't come to me when I wrote this rule. I still expected perfection, and I still demanded the best of myself. If other people didn't deliver perfection, that was okay! I didn't expect perfection from anyone except myself. Where this rule really began to have a new meaning was when I started to backslide in late December and early January. Backsliding after I wrote these 22 rules? How can that be? How can that happen? Backsliding, therefore was a mistake. This was a mistake that was threatening to unravel everything I did. Then for some reason, I figured out what was happening. I was beating myself up for beating myself up. I was beating myself up for allowing myself to regress and possibly go back to where I was before. This was a bad cycle and I had to put on the brakes. I had to get to a place where I could rationally work this out. If I didn't do something, I wasn't going to be able to get out of the hole. I had to make some drastic choices, not received well by all but they had to be made. I was letting other people and other events shape my own psyche. I had to get myself out of an environment where negativity and negative actions were fertile breeding ground for my period of regression. Some people didn't like the choices I made. Those some people were not in my head and didn't know what I was thinking. While this goes back to taking responsibility and taking a leadership role, that experience taught me a lot about what I was doing to myself.

Mistakes are a part of life. We all make them. We all must own up to them, yes. There are consequences to mistakes. Yet when I make a mistake I have to (sometimes force myself) look at it in a different light by asking some basic questions; Do I recognize what I did wrong?; Did I file this away for future reference?; How will I avoid doing this in the future? Once I answer these questions, I try to file it in the "done that" folder and move on. Lately, bowling and chess have been like that. After my last chess tournament, I put my games in the computer and reviewed the games I lost. What could I have done better? What did I miss? Instead of getting upset, I would note it and remember that for the next tournament. I will say that since I have made these drastic changes, I have had better results. Not perfect, but better. I still have moments where I feel like I am backsliding. I just have to stop and take stock. I try not to dwell so much any longer, and quite frankly I've been so busy that I don't have a lot of time to stew.

One of the things that is hanging on the wall in my living room is a shadowbox that contains the author copies of my first two books. The cover of A Patzer's Story is a human hand trying to keep a King from tipping over. In chess, the laying down of the King is a symbol of surrender or resignation, which ends the game. The symbolism is that I was showing in the cover that I was trying to keep myself from resigning the overall "game of life". Resignation from life, in my opinion is suicide. I don't know how many times I have just wanted it to "be done" so that I can have some peace. Resignation would have been the ultimate mistake, one that I certainly couldn't take back and one that I certainly couldn't learn from. I'm bound and determined not to make the last mistake. Let depression lose. Not me.

Rule 12: The only game you should play is on the chessboard

Again, I'm flexing my "literary license" muscle to take you down a somewhat different path that you may not expect, but this is a path that is worth exploring. Honestly I was having a bit of writer's block when starting this chapter, so I really had to step back and take a long look at this rule.

I wrote in <u>A Patzer's Story</u>, "Unless you're a Jedi Knight, don't play psychological games or tricks with your opponent". They will backfire. Also what can be said is don't let your opponent's games or tricks affect you. I have seen this on so many occasions, and at so many levels. Most of what I have seen has not even been at a chessboard. The sad part about this is that the effect of these games and tricks spilled over to innocent people. Even worse is that the people playing these games and tricks either didn't realize or didn't care how far reaching their actions were.

I've known people that were so vindictive that their response to anger or perceived injustice was revenge. I once knew a woman who told me that she was so upset at her (then) spouse that she cleaned the bathroom with his toothbrush, and laughed about it. I also knew a woman who was so narcissistic that she would always try to turn the attention to her, and throw a tantrum if it wasn't. She once got so upset at that, she burst out of a restaurant, sending a sign down one flight of stairs. She then acted as though nothing had happened. I realize that these are not the true form of psychological games or tricks, but it does illustrate how broad of a definition it is. I will be the first to admit that I engage in some form of "trash talking", especially at the bowling alley of late, but we all understand that it is done in jest. It helps to relax the tone, nobody gets hurt and we all shake hands afterward. That is one thing. What I described earlier though, is different. What I described earlier is downright destructive behavior. It should not be tolerated, but unfortunately it is. Using your spouse's toothbrush (Disclaimer: I was not on either side of this occurrence) to clean the bathroom is disgusting on all levels, not to mention a health hazard. Some may have found it funny, and unfortunately sided with the person. Bolting out of a restaurant and breaking a sign may raise a few eyebrows and provide some cannon fodder for later conversations, but it is childish. This is negativity at its finest, and is the antithesis of what this book is all about. It affects everyone around, and breeds even more negativity. This is why it is admittedly easy to say but difficult to practice not letting negativity affect you. People are going to be negative. You're going to run into that, perhaps even on a daily basis. It may be general negativity or directed at you. It is easy to ignore people that have general negative feelings, but how do you deal with negativity that is directed at you? First off, look at Rule 23, There is no such thing as a wrong feeling. This is important. It doesn't matter whether you agree or disagree with it. It just IS. You can choose to confront it, or ignore it and walk away. The choice is yours, and there is no wrong answer. It really depends on the situation, and the answer to this question - Is it really worth your time and energy to confront it? If you're going to confront it, make sure that there is something tangible to gain from your time and energy. Make sure it is worth the confrontation.

There is a common theme that is emerging and I would like to share it. Each human being is unique though I realize that it did not take rocket science to figure that out. What this means, though, is that each person may respond differently to a given situation. Remember in A Patzer's Story that I said if you show a chess position to ten Grandmasters, you are going to get ten different opinions on how to play the position unless it is an obvious forced situation. Earlier here I said that what is positive and negative is up to you. What one may find positive another may find negative. I also said that how you deal with it is also up to you. Just remember something else that I said, which is negativity on top of negativity does not yield positive.

I just went through a difficult divorce, and during the midst of it, it was suggested that I "play dirty". What would have been the purpose behind that? To win? To win what? Financial gain? I had to weigh the benefits against the costs. Before this was suggested to me, I vowed to strive to live by these rules every day, but there are more rules to be followed. Not only are there the legalistic rules but just the rules of integrity. When I was bowling the tournament in April I remember a particular frame in that on one of my spare shots, the ball bounced out of the gutter and actually picked up the spare. Now in the rules of bowling, the spare doesn't count. As I was working to correct the score, one of the people I was bowling with told me, "Just leave it". I thought otherwise. I'm going to strive to follow the rules. This was the tournament where I placed second, and that spare may have made the difference between first and second place. In spite of this I don't regret the decision that I made to correct the score and make it right. I didn't break the rules then, I didn't "play dirty" with my divorce.

The definition of "games" or "tricks" is pretty broad. We can talk about gamesmanship which I wrote about in A Patzer's

<u>Story</u>, but "games" or "tricks" can also mean someone who plays dirty, or someone who prefers to be negative; though it could be argued that playing dirty is also negative. Negativity is a recurring theme in this book because it has been something that I have had to deal with for a long time. Negative people, negative situations and my own negativity. Earlier I said that it boils down to basic math. A negative, when added to a negative, yields more negative. I will give one example; when I did poorly in a bowling tournament (negative) I would have a long car ride home and beat myself up (negative), which only fueled my downward spiral (more negative). Really, I was letting my mind play tricks on me by trying to convince me that I was worthless, didn't know what I was doing and the list goes on. So in the broader sense, it doesn't necessarily have to be another person or a situation. It could be your mind playing games with you. Remember that the human brain is the most complex organ we have in our system, and researchers haven't even begun to uncover the mysteries, though so much has been learned about it.

So how did I finally turn the corner? Truthfully, I'm not sure that I have turned the corner. I'm better at spotting the danger signs, and I'm getting better at keeping myself out of those situations. I'm trying not to let people or situations get into my head though sometimes it is unavoidable. The real challenge is to not let my brain play games with my psyche. It is relatively easy to ignore other people or situations. It is not so easy to ignore my own brain.

Rule 13: Win with grace, lose with dignity

Winning and losing is a part of everyday life. We compete for something every day, whether it is first or last in the checkout line, jockeying for position in traffic or grabbing the last available table in a crowded restaurant. Sometimes we win, and sometimes we lose. Sometime when we lose, we accept it and move on. Other times, we don't accept it and become very upset over this. The rule, in its original context had to do with head to head competition with other people but as I have learned in the last few months, it goes beyond that. For me, wins and losses also are related to my daily struggle with depression. I compete every day with forces that would serve to put me in a downward spiral, which include negativity and self-doubt. The deeper part of winning and losing is what you perceive in your mind as being a win or a loss.

While we can't win all the time, the real challenge for me is how I handle loss as it represents failure in some sort of way. I didn't win. I came up short. Once the outcome has been decided, we can't change it, and it is readily accepted most of the time. Since losing is negative, it breeds more negative. Where it becomes difficult for me is what happens afterward. I used to beat myself up, and was really good at it. It got to the point where after a loss or a not so good showing at a tournament, I would put myself in such a dwindling spiral that would take me days to recover. I piled negativity on more negativity to the point where I was even questioning a reason to get out of bed. Was this dignified? Not at all. Now don't get me wrong. I didn't lash out at anyone. All of my anger was directed inside, and not out. From outward appearances, I certainly was dignified, but internally I was not. While it is important to always act in a dignified manner to other people (Rule 7), it is more important to act in a dignified manner to yourself (Rule 7A).

I still struggle with losing. Whether at the chessboard, the bowling lane, work or whatever, I struggle with it. Yes, there is disappointment. It is a normal human reaction. We don't like to lose. There may be a little anger thrown in if the loss was due to a stupid mistake on my part. I contradict myself in this area, because mistakes are human and I forgive them when made by other people. I'm not so forgiving when I make them myself. Conversely, I don't expect people to be so forgiving to me, even though I can be more forgiving to other people. In other words, I don't hold people to the same standards that I hold myself to. In a way, that is fair, since everyone is different and has different values and beliefs. A lot of times though, that puts me in a losing position already as it leaves me vulnerable. Will I change this philosphy? Probably not, since it is a core value. But what I recently started doing and what has worked for me after a loss is the following checklist:

* What went right?
* What went wrong?
* How did the wrong cause the loss?
* What can I correct in the future?

Note that the FIRST item was "What went right?". While it is tough after being disappointed, I have to re-teach my mind to take the "glass half-full" attitude, and it is still a work in progress. I always try to preface something with a positive, if nothing else but to claim a win. "What went wrong?" is easy. What did I do wrong, followed by how did this cause the loss. Note that these tie in with rules 21 and 22 which will be covered later. When examining the "what went wrong" and "how did the wrong cause the loss" try and leave the emotion out of it.

Winning is a great feeling, no matter how small or insignificant the win may seem. It is positive, euphoric and sometimes adds a bounce to my step. Very recently, a reader of A Patzer's Story posted a wonderful review of the book. I was almost in tears when I read it. What a great win for me. We all feel good about a win, and rightfully so. It is also human nature to share the win with others as well. "Win with grace" means exactly that, though. Don't let the euphoria get out of hand. Avoid comments like "I kicked his butt", "We smoked 'em" or anything like that which can be disparaging. This is akin to "rubbing their nose" in it, and there is nothing positive about that. Conversely, there is a lot of positive to be able to recognize and celebrate even the smallest of wins. Sometimes just getting out of bed was a win for me. If I were to add an addendum to this rule, it would be "There is no such thing as a wrong win". Why? Because it is up to us to decide what a win really is. It's hard for me to pull even the smallest wins out of the biggest of disappointments. I recently bowled my first PBA tournament in about a year. I started out okay, but went downhill. Needless to say, after the tournament I was disappointed. While I didn't beat myself up as bad as I normally would have, which in itself was a win, I could have bowled better. I did objectively look at the mistakes I made, and am trying to correct them.

It is difficult for me to "unlearn" a behavior. For many years, I have had such a low self-esteem that I had to be the best at everything that I did. I always strived to be at the top, meaning that I always had to win. To not win was failure. To not be the "go to" guy, to not be the top in everything that I did was failure. Losing is still hard to swallow sometimes, but it also took me a long time to realize that my worth as a person was not decided by how many wins I have under my belt. It also took a long time for me to realize that losing, while negative does not constitute failure. Sometimes, even recognizing the smallest of wins can be the difference between a positive outlook and total despair.

Let's take a step back and put this in the simplest of persopectives that we can all agree on. Winning is great and losing sucks. If you win you're elated and if you lose you're deflated. Lately though, I have had recent experiences where I have had to put winning and losing in perspective and really look at the overall impact. This is another approach which has really helped me minimize the effect of a loss and put wins into another 'plane' if you will. Is the win a goal or merely a means to an end? What is the end result? Is it about winning? Is it about 'being right'? Sometimes I get so consumed with winning that I forget about the end goal, which may not at all be about winning anything. There is a saying that goes, "It's not about whether you win or lose, it's how you play the game". After a win, big or small, we can handle ourselves fairly well. Sometimes though I am so focused on the win and winning in the future that my mind gets clouded and the real end goal becomes fuzzy. Thus when I lose, I become even more deflated. So it boils down to this. When you win, celebrate but don't become consumed. When you lose, look at the big picture. Was it really a loss or a minor setback? Keep the wins and losses in perspective and don't lose sight of the end goal.

Rule 14: Leave your emotions outside the tournament room

I'm not a Vulcan, which means that I have emotions. For many years, I have held these emotions in check. I have been, and still am somewhat reluctant to display my emotions, which for many years I took as a sign of weakness. I've been in situations where display of emotions was highly discouraged. I had to be "the rock", the solid, stable base that everyone could lean on. Too much leaning made me tired and emotionally weak and also, in my opinion, fueled my depression. I'm not blaming anyone but me for that because I allowed it to happen. I own that and I will take responsibility for it.

When I wrote the rule, the context was to not show any emotion that might give your opponent a tip that there is something amiss on a chessboard. It goes back to an old TV commercial that said, "don't let them see you sweat". In other words, if you make that bad move, don't display any sort of outward expression that may tip your opponent off. While this is a valid guideline, I've learned over the last several months that there is a time to express emotions or 'get things off your chest', and there are times when this is not appropriate. Reviewing this rule made me really sit down and reflect. In my younger days, I had a very explosive temper. I wasn't violent to others, but violent to inanimate objects. Walls, doors, furniture and other objects were constant victims. As I grew up I was cautioned that I shouldn't do things like that, but I had no other outlet. Hence I kept a lot of things just bottled up. Keeping it inside was just as bad as hitting walls. I'm not saying that hitting doors is the answer. Destructive outlets are dangerous, and unacceptable if they are directed at people or animals. The other end of the spectrum though, keeping it bottled up is just as bad. So where is the happy medium? I think that this is up to the individual. We know how much we can handle without exploding and it differs from person to person. It is being able to recognize the breaking point and doing something constructive to "empty the bottle" before the bottle breaks. This is another area I still struggle with, as well as when it is appropriate to show and express emotions. Whatver you choose and whatever your limitations are, please avoid destructive behavior and violence against other people and animals. This is beyond negative. Don't drown your emotions in a bottle, regardless of whether it contains pills or alcohol. There is also nothing positive about this. If you feel as though you're going to hurt yourself or others or if you think you have an issue with substance abuse, will you please reach out to someone and get help?

I realize that I went off on a tangent here. While it is a good guideline to "leave your emotions outside the tournament room", it is not license to forget that you have them or to ignore them.

Rule 15: Make your opponent EARN the win

I think that there may be some contradictions in this section. I really had to step back and think about this rule, as I have with all the others. At first glance it makes sense. Don't resign, don't give up on a bad position, don't give up the ship; these are all still valid guidelines. In retrospect though, when I wrote <u>A Patzer's Story</u>, I admit that I had my blinders on and that I wrote it with somewhat of a narrow focus, which was on chess. I really had no idea how widespread these rules would become once I really started focusing on them. I thought about all the chess games that I have played, all the bowling tournaments that I have participated in, and all the other times I was in a 'win or lose' situation. While Rule #15 certainly applies to chess, bowling and other games or sports, there are other times in a 'win or lose' situation where a loss can be disastrous.

There are some opponents that you absolutely don't want to lose to. We all have challenges, or opponents if you will. No matter how we refer to them, whether 'demons', 'skeletons' or other types of names, they are still opponents because they are competing against you. I've had friends of mine who have had cancer, and they certainly considered cancer to be their opponent. If their opponent had beaten them, my friends would no longer be here. I've stated often that depression is my opponent and vowed that I would never let it beat me.

Some sports and games are meant to be 'individual' in

nature. Chess, golf and bowling are like that, as opposed to team sports such as football or baseball where you play a specific role on the team. With individual sports and games, you are responsible for your performance. In many situations you cannot have any sort of coaching and you can't go to the sidelines or the dugout. Those are the rules and they have to be followed. What about these other opponents though? What about these demons and skeletons? I definitely could not hold my own against them. This is where coaching and assistance is absolutely necessary. I did touch on this briefly in my first book, and I will expand on it here. For me to get through my depression, coaching and advice was and still is absolutely necessary. In chess or bowling, I would sometimes lose, but life goes on. Depression, at least for me, is not a game nor is it a sport. I didn't realize until about a year ago how serious it really was. It is something that I don't want to lose to.

Don't resign. Don't concede defeat. There is always something to gain out of any situation, no matter how hopeless it may seem. Anytime you can learn or gain something, even in the worst of situations is a positive, which is really a win.

**Rule 16: Your coach knows more about chess than you do,
Rule 17: You learn more when your eyes and ears are open,
Rule 18: You learn less when your mouth is open,
Rule 19: There is no such thing as a stupid question**

If someone told me that they don't need any coaching, they are only kidding themselves. I personally don't know everything about everything. I've been bowling for over 30 years, and I still don't understand some of the nuances of the game, especially the technology that is becoming commonplace with new equipment. I certainly don't know everything about chess, because I still learn something from each of my games. These are reasons that I have worked with chess coaches and bowling coaches. I want to improve, I want to learn something from somebody who is familiar with what I need to learn more about. It's about keeping my pride and ego in check and saying that I need help. I had to do this when I was at the low point. I had to leave my pride and ego at home, walk into a therapist's office and say, "I need help".

A good coach will take the time to assess your strengths and weaknesses. A good coach may even uncover weaknesses that you never thought you had. The key is to trust them and let them do their job. I know a few people who have had coaching in various situations, and the first time they sit with their coach, they are telling the coach all that they know, plus all the reasons that they won't do what the coach wants them to do. I've seen this in group therapy as well as other situations. I also used to be this way, but I found out the hard way that it doesn't work. It didn't work for chess, it didn't work for bowling and it certainly didn't work in therapy. I had to swallow my pride as well as my ego, leave it at home and walk into therapy in a very vulnerable state. It wasn't comfortable at all and some parts were just unpleasant. Nonetheless I had to sit there and keep my mouth shut, which I did by choice and not coercion. I had to trust my coaches, knowing that they had the degrees and certifications in mental health, while I did not. I had to listen to what they said, no matter how unpleasant it made me feel. Nevertheless, I did this willingly because I really had no other alternative. It was at my lowest point when I realized that what I was doing at the time wasn't really working for me, and that I needed to drastically change my approach. My pride and my ego were getting in the way of my mental health, so some of my priorities had to be reset. This was a difficult process. After all, I was a senior consultant where I was working. I was used to coaching other people, and now here I need coaching myself. I had to admit to myself that I had serious issues that needed to be handled and that I couldn't do it alone.

I still to this day sometimes have difficulty with my ego and my pride. I'm seeing a therapist for ongoing maintenance, and at times it is difficult to admit that I still have issues, even after baring some of my soul in print as I have done with my previous books. It is sometimes hard to face that there are some issues that I am going to have for the rest of my life. There are still many things that I am working through. As I have said before and I will say again, I am a work in progress. Depression is a lifelong struggle, and there are still some areas about me that need to be looked at, evaluated and possibly modified. I can't do this alone, and I need help doing it.

Rule 20: Don't let anyone rain on your parade

There have been many times in my life where I have achieved the biggest of wins, only to be deflated by something or someone that is negative. A negative comment, a negative situation or even something as simple as someone totally ignoring the accomplishment. It's truly a deflating moment. I would put in a lot of work to accomplish something huge, and it is minimized to the point where I and my accomplishment would feel like nothing. I have struggled with this dilemma for many years. Earlier I wrote about effort, in Rule #3. You get out what you put in. I would put in all of this work, all of this effort and achieve a major milestone. Then, nobody seemed to care what I did. Oftentimes, not only would the milestone be ignored but my faults would be spotlighted, or just be told "Okay, now go and do this…". I don't think anything can be more deflating to a person's soul and mood more than this type of reaction or lack of reaction.

This is a tough struggle for me. Acceptance is a basic human need, and I would feel as though I wasn't getting any acceptance or acknowledgement. After a while, I would put in the effort but it would be more 'going through the motions' knowing that my efforts would be unnoticed or minimized. Knowing or feeling that there was no brass ring would leave me with an empty feeling and questioning my own value and worth. This is where the downward spiral begins. Questioning my own value and self-worth was a major contributor to my depression, as I felt that I didn't have anything of value to offer the world. If I felt that I wasn't of any value, what is my purpose and what good am I doing here? Does this sound familiar? It is very familiar to me, and to this day I still struggle with it. Today though, I have found a great group of people who are fellow authors, work colleagues and other people who are positive and keep my spirits lifted.

The keys in my struggle with this are acceptance and acknowledgement. I wanted people to acknowledge what I accomplished, and be accepted. If I didn't get one or the other, my effort was for naught and my own perception of my worth was diminished. In reality, my deeper struggle was my perception of my own self-worth, which also went hand-in-hand with my self-esteem. Both my own self-worth and self-esteem were lacking. These were areas that needed serious work. Actually, these are areas that still need work. I can still hear voices in my past telling me that I am useless and worthless. There are days when I can't hear the voices but there are days when the voices are loud and clear. This rang so true recently when someone posted an anonymous review of one of my books. The review itself was inaccurate and laced with personal attacks, but I couldn't help but hear the voices when I read that. This is a prime example of not only minimizing an accomplishment, but also responding to it with fault. I couldn't help but feel deflated, and questioning my motivation for publishing the book in the first place. So how did I counter this? First off I had to recognize that this was only one person out of many, and someone who obviously didn't read the book. I had to consider the source of the negativity. Second, I had to reaffim my own worth by reminding myself of why I wrote the book in the first place and also reminding myself that the anonymous reviewer was not my publisher.

Finally, and this is something that took a little time, the people that have read any enjoyed my book far outnumbered this one lone person. I did touch another person's life by sharing my struggles. I did do something positive.

I often struggle with the realization that my worth is not measured by what other people think about me. It is what I think about myself. While the opinions of others do certainly count, it is my opinion of myself that matters the most. With that, I have to make sure that I still have some measure of humility and not over-inflate my ego. It has to be kept in perspective. Humility is something that I don't have a problem with, because I know that I am far from perfect and I make more than my share of mistakes. Conversely I also make my share of accomplishments.While a lot of these accomplishments and milestones are often not recognized or even minimized, I still accomplished something. I finally have the sense to carry an umbrella, because there is always someone out there who will try to rain on my parade.

Rule 21: You must be able to OBJECTIVELY face your current limitations

In the last chapter, I wrote about having humility while knowing that I am worth something. I wrote about the need to caution myself over overestimating my self-worth. Knowing and accepting that I am far from perfect is quite easy. Beating myself up over falling short of goals and realizations is also very easy for me. I have previously wrote that when it comes to beating myself up, I am an expert. I do that quite well, even though this was counterproductive to any path I needed to take to get better. This is still a struggle for me at times, especially when there was a lot of emotional and mental investment in the effort. The emotional effort is a difficult thing to discount since it was part of the effort but it also is a hindrance when trying to determine what went wrong. Go back to what I wrote in rule #13, especially when evaluating what went wrong. It is important to be able to leave the emotion out of the evaluation and OBJECTIVELY, which means without emotion and without pre-conceived opinion, come face to face with what went wrong. With emotion, my reaction would be, "I'm really horrible. I have no business being here!". There is no objectivity to this. Without emotion, my reaction would be something like, "I moved that Knight too early" or "Hand position wasn't right. The lanes were changing too quick and I couldn't read them". Note the difference? Analyzing without emotion allows you to get more to the root cause of the issue. An excellent example of this is the person that I work for today. Very recently we had some challenges on the project that I was working on. These challenges were threatening to put the entire project behind schedule. My manager, instead of pointing fingers and trying to place blame, very calmly said, "What can we do to fix this?". Without emotion, we came up with a plan and the plan was successful. Hence we were able to keep our project on track and on schedule. It is people like Jeanne who epitomize this rule and live the rule day to day. Not only that, but Jeanne also epitomizes the other rules in this book as well. She is a person who sets a true example of what is right in this world.

Rule #14 also applies here. Leave your emotions outside the tournament room, and also leave your emotions outside the evaluation process. Admittedly, it is easier said than done. Lately, the approach I use is to not do the evaluation right after the event. I would wait and let my emotion subside as well as letting myself "chill out" after the event. To me this is important. it gives me an opportunity to 'wind down' so that when I finally get to the evalutation phase, I'm not so pent up with emotion and mental thoughts swirling around my head. In other words I try to have a clear head.

The other challenge I have in this area is how much 'nit-picking' is actually necessary. It is very easy for me to find my own faults (and there are many) but how many of these faults are real vs. perceived or objective vs. subjective. Even when I leave the emotion out of it, the subjective faults sometimes sneak into the evaluation. This is finding even the smallest of faults, event when the fault had nothing to do with the result. "I was wearing the wrong shirt", or things of that nature. This is very easy for me to do. When I add to the list of faults, it is difficult to even think about how to correct them. As the list of 'what went wrong' grows longer, it becomes more difficult to see light at the end of the tunnel. Hence, correcting the faults seems to be an overwhelming task. To combat this I have to sit down and consider what really went wrong. My shirt had nothing to do with it. My move sequence, or the bad decision I made with respect to choice of equipment could well have had a lot to do with it.

In life outside of chess and bowling, the ability to objectively face limitations is even more important. It is tough to transition from "I am worthless" to "I am worth something". To be able to objectively list my faults without having the list in multiple volumes to fill the Library of Congress is tough. To be able to list my strengths as well as my faults was even more of a challenge.

Rule 22: You must always celebrate and embrace your strengths

There were days when I woke up in the morning and wonder why I even bothered. There were days when I would go through the motions, doing only enough to get through the day. There were days when I felt worthless and incompetent. I still have these days sometimes but not as often as before. I try to wake up each morning with an attitude that I have strengths and I do have something to offer the world. In a serious, depressive state this is a tough challenge. In a depressive state it is very easy to list my limitations and very tough to list my strengths.

Go back to Rule #13 for a moment when I talked about the 'glass half-full' attitude. Even the smallest wins should be celebrated with grace. Even the smallest strengths should be embraced, each and every day. No matter how obscure it may be, celebrate it and embrace it. It is yours and nobody can take it away from you. There is an exercise that I do when I am in a depressed state. Let me share it with you. When you first do this, try to allow about five minutes in a quiet place with no interruptions. Ignore your phone, your email and any other interruptions you may encounter.

Once you have settled in, consider your current mood. Make note of it on a scale of one to 10 with one being the lowest and 10 being the highest. Then for the next five minutes, think about your strengths and write them down. Feel free to photocopy the page titled 'MY STRENGTHS' and use it. I am doing this mentally now, but as you are doing this exercise for the first few times you will want to write them down.

What qualifies as a strength? Anything positive that you can think about yourself. No matter how blase or mundane, write it down. Be as generous as you like. Remember that there is no such thing as a wrong feeling (Rule #23). At first you may not be able to fill the page though I would challenge you to do so. After the five minutes, review what you wrote down and consider what your mood is. Take note of it and compare it to your mood before the exercise. Is it higher? It should be. As we start thinking better of ourselves, we start being more positive. Try to do this at least once a day. Repeating what you wrote the previous day is not only allowed but strongly encouraged. After all, a strength that you have today will certainly be with you tomorrow. An optional step to this exercise is to keep these 'logs' in a journal of some sort. Review them over a period of time to see if you are listing more strengths each day and if your overall mood is getting better.

Remember that perception of worth doesn't start with your friends, family, acquaintences or associates. It starts with you. You are responsible not only for your own development, but for your own thoughts and attitude. While it may seem harsh and egotistic to say. "to hell with what other people think", sometimes we have to take that attitude in order to start getting better. I know I had to. When I was in therapy I encountered a few people who talked about things that triggered memories from my past. What they talked about, I cannot divulge but what they said really hit home for me and gave me the impression that I was worthless. I was like that for a day or so until I realized that I wasn't in therapy for them. I was in it for me. So basically I had to adopt the attitude that everyone else except my doctors and therapists can go to hell because

I needed to get better. Arrogant? Certainly. Of course I would participate in therapy and give constructive output when I could, but at the end of the day I had to take responsibility for getting better. That meant I had to take what other people said and let it slide off my back.

I'm not by nature an arrogant person. I respect and value the opinions of those close to me, and I seek counsel from those friends when I need it. I always know that there are a few people who not only will give me their honest opinion but they will also do it in such a way that is positive. These are people, though, that know me and know where I have been. I know that what they have to say is from the heart and yet they still value me as a person. I'm not above criticism. Anyone who knows me well will acknowledge that. But back in the days of my therapy and for some time thereafter, I had to keep the arrogant attitude. While I keep it in check today, it still comes out at times, for example when that horrible review was posted. I basically had to say "to hell with this person" and move on. It did take a couple of days for me to get over that review - which is still posted and sometimes it does bother me - but when I look at the number of posittive reviews it makes me feel better. Yes I am gaining my strength from others, but sometimes I have to lean on that in order to get my positive psyche kick-started.

Sometimes I was in such a depressed state that I didn't even believe my own affirmations of worthiness. It is hard to believe something good about myself when I was so low to the ground. Sometimes I needed a "kick-start" and some of the people in my therapy group, including my therapist were great at giving me the kick start. While this may seem like it goes against the axiom that it doesn't matter what other people think, it is important to note that especially when it comes to my own mental health, I can't go it alone. I need to have some people in my own corner willing to cheer me on and give me a lift when I need it. But while their opinions are important, it is mine that matters the most because when I list those strengths, those are coming from me and my heart.

Feel free to reproduce as many copies of this page as you wish.

MY STRENGTHS

Date:

Mood Before (1 - 10 with 1 being the worst and 10 being the best):

Mood After (1 - 10 with 1 being the worst and 10 being the best):

Now here comes the tough question. Do you actually believe, and I mean truly believe without a doubt what you wrote down? Think about that for a minute? Did you write them down because you truly believe it or because you want to believe it? Do you really think and believe that you have compassion or is that what you are striving to be? **Celebrating and embracing your strengths requires belief in yourself.** When I wrote <u>A Patzer's Story</u> I had no delusions that it would hit the bestseller list or win a Pulitzer Prize. I wrote it to touch lives, but I didn't know and couldn't gauge to what extent it would. There were ups and downs, and days when I questioned my own ability as an author. But one day, very recently, a reader posted a review on my Facebook page. A very touching review that left me speechless. One thing it did do was fuel my belief in myself. Sometimes we do need that external affirmation, but when you do celebrate your strengths by writing them down, take a moment and answer this question; "Do I really believe this about me?". If you don't, find your coach.

I ran across this poem by fellow author Debbie Hunt, and she graciously allowed me to reprint it here. This is the perfect way to close this chapter of the book.

EMBRACE

Embrace yourself with trust and appreciation

Embrace life with hope and fascination

Embrace the journey with peace and realization

Embrace friendship with fun and admiration

Embrace children with joy and adoration

Embrace love with excitement and devotion

Embrace every moment~

Embrace all there is.

Rule 23: There is no such thing as a wrong feeling

First off, I need to repeat the disclaimer that I am not a mental health professional, nor do I have any degrees or certifications in this area. Everything that I wrote in all of my books thus far are based on my own personal experience, with my own personal observations and opinions mixed in. Whether or not you agree with everything I write is solely up to you. Your opinions and feelings after you have read one or all of my books are solely up to you.

Our early experiences shape our belief and value systems. These beliefs and values shape the way that we feel or react to certain situations. Some reactions are reflex reactions. Not 'knee-jerk' but totally reflex. For example, if someone is taking a swing at me, my initial reaction is to either put up my guard to block the swing or to move so that the person would miss the swing. This is a reaction. A feeling is different. What would I feel? Anger, maybe fear, maybe I would feel ready for a fight. Who knows? A person who has a belief system that places a high value on non-violence may still get out of the way, but not have the feelings of anger. This person, based on their belief system may feel pity toward the attacker. So who is right? Who is wrong? The answer is we are both right. I may go to the other person who was attacked and ask why he won't fight back or defend himself, and I may get a response that he is a believer in non-violence and doesn't feel the anger that I do. We are both right, but that does not give me license to tell him, "You shouldn't feel that way. He just tried to hit you". The worst words you can ever say to a person is, "You shouldn't feel that way". This will invalidate their entire belief system, and serve to demoralize them. Also you risk alienation, and withdrawal is dangerous especially if the person is in a depressed state.

On the flip side of this is your own feelings. I and I alone am responsible for the way I feel, and I am also responsible for any consequences that may result from the way I feel. In the previous example, if I felt anger and decided to fight back, I am responsible for the consequences of that conflict. Your reaction to a certain situation may be governed by reflex, but your feelings afterward are completely within your control. Recently I received a somewhat nasty email that made me very angry. I responded to it in kind, which made for an even nastier response. Essentially what I did was pile negativity on top of negativity which was wrong on my part. While the second response was even nastier, when I saw that, I also saw the error of my ways. I accepted responsibility and wrote a much nicer response to the email which of course, included an apology. Feelings, and the subsequent actions afterward can either defuse or escalate a situation. I have to work to keep my feelings in check such that they don't produce the negativity that I recently made the mistake of doing.

You cannot be responsible for what someone else feels, and nobody else can be responsible for what you feel. I've often run into situations where the other person said, "You made me feel that way". What did I do to cause the other person to feel a certain way? Again, feelings are shaped by our values and belief system. I used to blame other people for the way that I would feel, but I had to step back and take a look at where the feelings were coming from. We can no more accept responsibility for what another person feels than we can have others accept responsibility for the way we feel. Once I accepted that responsibility I could better gauge where my feelings were coming from and why, once they were not all blurred by finger pointing. Finger pointing, or in more politically correct prose, deflection of blame is an attempt to 'run away' from one's feelings and not accept responsibility. Saying "you made me feel this way" can bring up feelings of guilt and possibly misguided responsibility. Tack that on to negativity, and there is certainly no good in that.

What's the bottom line here? People have a right to feel what they want to feel and we should accept responsibility for what we feel.

Rule 24: A little discomfort is necessary to achieve the desired result

Over the last few months, I have been suffering with arthritis in both of my shoulders. This was diagnosed some time ago, but recently became almost unbearable. As it turned out, I had a herniated disc in my neck. After getting a referral to another doctor (and another doctor after that), I started to get cortisone injections. The first injection was in the shoulder which was not bad, and provided some releif. But after a few weeks, the pain was still there so a decision was made to do a series of injections in my neck where the disc was in order to releive the pressure on the nerve. A needle in my neck that close to my spinal cord???? Every horrible thought went through my head. What if the needle nicked the cord? What if I flinched during the injection? Needless to say I was more than a little anxious. At the first appointment, I was taken into one of their procedure rooms that had a state of the art X-ray machine, which the doctor used to do a very precision injection. Laying on my side on the table, the doctor and his assistant were very reassuring and his assistant even acknowledged that the position I was laying in, combined with the proper positioning for the injection was uncomfortable. In order to feel better, I had to do this. I had to "suck up" the discomfort. Needless to say, the injection was relatively painless and the doctor of course performed with his usual brilliancy. But laying on my side with a needle being stuck in my neck and the discomfort of the cortisone being injected into my neck was where I thought of this rule.

Reflecting on this, it was also during therapy where I had to go through a lot of discomfort in order to acheive the desired result. I had to reflect on my past, and come to terms with a lot of misconceptions that I have held about myself through the years. Therapy was very uncomfortable for me as I had to come to terms with a lot of suppressed feelings. I had to let go of a lot of misconceptions about myself, and pretty much lay myself bare at times. There were a lot of tears, some anger, some frustration, a lot of anxiety and a lot of sad moments. But I never lost hope that there is light at the end of a long dark tunnel that spanned 40 plus years. No matter how long and dark the tunnel may seem, I always had the hope that there would be a light at the end so that I can continue my journey. A Patzer's Journey.

Final Thoughts

I am by no means cured of depression. No matter what anyone says, depression is a life long struggle. Today I am managing it through medication and therapy. I don't see a therapist as often as I did before, because I feel today that I only need to check in every so often but my therapist is available should I have a crisis, a breakdown or a regression. Help is always a phone call away. I am by no means a perfect person. You may think, "Wow. He has his act together". While I thank you for that compliment, I still have struggles today. These are struggles that are not insurmountable but struggles nonetheless. I don't let these struggles overwhelm me, because there are other aspects of my life that are going reasonably well. But we all have struggles of one form or another. There are days when I wish that I could just leave my struggles behind. It reminds me of the time when I used to travel a lot. Compared to most people that traveled, I think that I overpacked. I would see people with the little wheeled carry on and a computer bag. Me? A suitcase, a small bag and my computer bag. That's a lot of baggage to drag around. Over the years, we accumulate a lot of stuff. Even after living in my apartment for a few months, I seem to have accumulated a lot. Today it is a far cry from what I had a few months ago. I also have accumulated a lot of mental baggage. Reminders of my past, some good and some bad. I can't erase memories, nor is it possible to leave them behind. It isn't possible to ignore my struggles as they won't go away. The best I can do today is to embrace what I have, which is the ability to write and a strong desire to touch people's lives in a positive manner. I have touched many lives with <u>A Patzer's Story</u> and it is my heartfelt wish to touch yours with this book.

Just a reminder that this book is not a 'cookbook' and it is not intended to be something that will cure you of all your ailments. I've written what has worked for me, based on my personal experiences, observations and opinions. As they say in some commercials, "Your mileage may vary". Toward the end of the book is a separate page listing the 24 rules. Feel free to make a copy of this page if there are rules that mean anything at all to you. Tape them to your mirror, make an index card or copy them to your computer. All I ask of you is that if the rules make sense to you, please do your best to live by them on a daily basis.

Thank you for taking the time to read my book. You can reach me at <u>tsawyer@mbdsolus.com</u>. Enjoy your journey.

Acknowledgements

Over the last several months I have made friendships with some wonderful people. These relationships are both in person and online, and without their support it would have been more difficult to publish my books. There are a few people that stand out, and I want to give them a special mention here.

Where would I be without fellow authors Shannon Clark and Debbie Hunt? Both are profound writers as well as wonderful people. They both took time from their own writing and families to help with reviewing and proofreading. More important, their moral support and friendship has been beyond valuable. Thank you both.

To Laura; she proofread, opined, proofread and opined multiple times. Her friendship, candor, intelligence and support are valuable to me. We had some very profound discussions about rule #23, and gave me a perspective that I never considered before. She has been a constant supporter and her friendship as well as her insight is also valuable.

Jeanne, what can I say? In only a few short months she has earned my deep respect as well as becoming a close friend.

To my friends on Facebook, you know who you are. You're always a source of positive inspiration. Whenever the chips seem to be down, you always do something to make me smile or laugh. Some of my friends are authors, but I also want to give a special 'thank you' to my classmates from Branham High School, '81.

To my family; Mom, Elaine, Kathy and David as well as my nieces and nephews.

To Dad; if he were alive today, I'm not sure if there would be anyone prouder. But I know that with each book published and each book sold, he celebrates.

And finally, but certainly not least, there is Wendy. My nine-pound, four-legged, canine editor-in-chief didn't contribute a lot of editorial content, but that wasn't important to me. She has a heart full of unconditional love that she freely gives. It's surprising what one can learn from a dog.

Feel free to reproduce as many copies of this page as you wish.

The Rules

Rule 1: There is no "magic bullet" or "magic pill" that will make you a grandmaster (GM) overnight

Rule 2: You must accept responsibility for your own game and development

Rule 3: What you get out of chess is directly proportional to the effort that you put in

Rule 4: Your opponent is human

Rule 5: Your opponent is out to win and will give you a tough fight

Rule 6: A rating is only a number

Rule 7: Treat your opponent as you want to be treated

Rule 7A: Treat yourself as you want to be treated

Rule 8: Any plan is better than no plan

Rule 9: You may have a plan but your opponent has one too

Rule 10: No plan survives the next move

Rule 11: A chess game is won by the player who makes the NEXT to last mistake

Rule 12: The only game that you should be playing is on the chessboard

Rule 13: Win with grace, lose with dignity

Rule 14: Leave your emotions outside the tournament room

Rule 15: Make your opponent EARN the win

Rule 16: Your coach knows more about chess than you do

Rule 17: You learn more when your eyes and ears are open

Rule 18: You learn less when your mouth is open

Rule 19: There is no such thing as a stupid question

Rule 20: Don't let anyone rain on your parade

Rule 21: You must be able to objectively face your current limitations

Rule 22: You must always celebrate and embrace your strengths
Rule 23: There is no such thing as a wrong feeling
Rule 24: A little discomfort is necessary to acheive the desired result

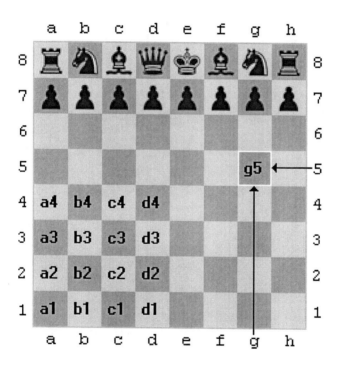

Chess Notation

In the game that was shown earlier in the book, this is known as algebraic notation. This is the simple form of chess notation that is now widely used. Each chess square has a letter and corresponding number, as shown in the board below. At the start of the game, the White pieces occupy rows 1 & 2 while the Black pieces occupy rows 3 & 4.

To illustrate the first few moves in the game:
1.d4 Nf6 -> White moved the pawn from the d2 square to the d4 square. Black moved the Knight at g8 to the square on f6

2.c4 e6 3.g6 -> White moved the pawn on c2 to c4. Black moved the pawn on g7 to g6

3 Bb4+ 4.Nd7 -> White moved the Bishop on f1 to the b4 square, giving check (noted by the +sign). Black responded by placing the Knight on f6 to the d7 square

Using the notation and a chessboard, it is easy to replay a game that is recorded in algebraic notation. Those interested in learning more can visit the US Chess Federation website at http://www.uschess.org.

Books by Timothy A. Sawyer and Other Favorite Authors

Both of my previous books are available through my publisher, PublishAmerica (http://www.publishamerica.com), my website (http://www.authorsden.com/timothysawyer) as well as major booksellers in the United States and around the world. They are available in softcover as well as 'E-Book' format. If you have a problem locating any of my books, please drop me a note at tsawyer@mbdsolus.com, and I will be more than happy to help.

A Patzer's Story (PublishAmerica, 2010) ISBN-13: 978-1-4560-3797-0

My Email to God Bounced (PublishAmerica, 2011) ISBN-13: 978-1-4560-5627-8

Also, please consider books from a few of my favorite author friends.

Wollie the Wheelbarrow by Debbie Colleen Hunt (PublishAmerica, 2011). Author's note: This book is in pre-release, but Debbie is on Facebook. Debbie is the author of the poem Embrace, featured earlier in this book.

Quilochet by Shannon Clark (PublishAmerica, 2011) ISBN-13: 978-1-4560-7072-4

Ashi's Gift by Anne Eskeldson (PublishAmerica, 2011) ISBN-13: 978-1-4560-1761-3

Longing for December by Sheila Shaffer-Burket (PublishAmerica, 2011). *Author's note: This book is in pre-release, but Shelia is on Facebook.*

Coming soon…

Jan "Jesse" Schild is trying to rebuild his life after a drug lab linked to the Nikitin drug cartel explodes, killing his wife and daughter. After moving halfway across the country to get away from the memories, he once again confronts his nemesis, who threatens another innocent person. Jesse vows that Nikitin will get to nobody else while he is drawing breath. Jesse has an unknown ally in the person of Sgt. Frank Price, who heads a multi-jurisdiction drug task force. Frank has been chasing Nikitin for going on 10 years. Does the Nikitin cartel finally collapse?

<u>Trip Four</u> by Timothy A. Sawyer

CPSIA information can be obtained
at www.ICGtesting.com
Printed in the USA
FFOW021320051212
374FF